Managing Joint Pain

How to Control Arthritis

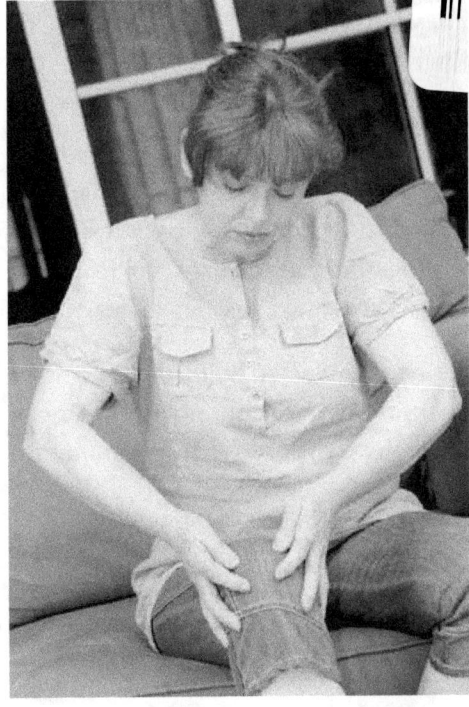

Natural Health Series

Dueep J Singh

Mendon Cottage Books

JD-Biz Publishing

Disclaimer

The information is this book is provided for informational purposes only. It is not intended to be used and medical advice or a substitute for proper medical treatment by a qualified health care provider. The information is believed to be accurate as presented based on research by the author.

The contents have not been evaluated by the U.S. Food and Drug Administration or any other Government or Health Organization and the contents in this book are not to be used to treat cure or prevent disease.

The author or publisher is not responsible for the use or safety of any diet, procedure or treatment mentioned in this book. The author or publisher is not responsible for errors or omissions that may exist.

Warning

The Book is for informational purposes only and before taking on any diet, treatment or medical procedure, it is recommended to consult with your primary health care provider.

Check out some of the other Healthy Gardening Series books at Amazon.com

Gardening Series on Amazon

Check out some of the other Health Learning Series books at Amazon.com

Health Learning Series on Amazon

Table of Contents

Introduction

Many people are confused when they come across terms like arthritis and rheumatism. According to the Mayo Clinic, arthritis is the medical term for joint pain. Rheumatism is muscular pain brought about by inflammation and infection in the muscular tissues.

Did you know that about 52 million people in the USA alone are suffering from some sort of arthritis, or joint pain? Most of them have a feeling that this is one of the occupational hazards, which one has to bear the moment one starts getting old. But that is not necessarily true.

Arthritis can be caused due to any injury or to some disease than is going to include pain, stiffness and swelling. It can hit you at any age, especially when the joint has got inflamed. Inflammation is the body's natural reaction to any portion of the body which has undergone some sort of muscular tissue trauma due to injury or infection.

Arthritis is going to affect the musculoskeletal system of your body, especially the joints. This is then going to cause slow and steady disability and stiffness, and people over the age of 50 are more vulnerable to such problems.

Types of Arthritis

There are two very common types of arthritis recognized by experienced medical practitioners. These are rheumatoid arthritis and osteoarthritis. Osteoarthritis is the more common type of arthritis of the two. This normally affects the joints around bones, and it is going to come with age. It affects the knees and the hips.

Puma tired. Arthritis occurs when your immunity system is not working in a healthy fashion. It is going to affect your bones and the joints, often affecting those joints in your feet and in your hands. It may also affect your internal system and organs.

Symptoms of Arthritis

You know that you are going to be suffering from arthritis in the future, when you begin to feel fatigue and fever in the initial stages. Then signs of joint inflammation are going to include tenderness, warmth, swelling, pain, stiffness and redness in that particular area.

These symptoms are going to vary from person to person, depending on the infection or upon the severity of the inflammation.

During this time, one or more joints are going to be inflamed, possibly because of the spreading of the infection. This is going to limit the normal healthy day to day functioning of your joints.

Arthritis is not restricted to one particular age group, anybody can suffer from it. Even children suffer from arthritis, especially when it has been caused due to some injury or some tissue trauma.

Women are considered to be more vulnerable to arthritis, when compared to men. 60% of the arthritis patients about the age of 50 are women.

Arthritis is going to start with some pain in some portion of your body. Pain is the way which your body tells you that something is wrong with your tissues or muscles. This pain can lead to stiffness, fatigue, discomfort and swelling in that particular portion. This is later going to lead to disability and deformity, though that does not happen in all cases. Many of the arthritis cases are self-limiting.

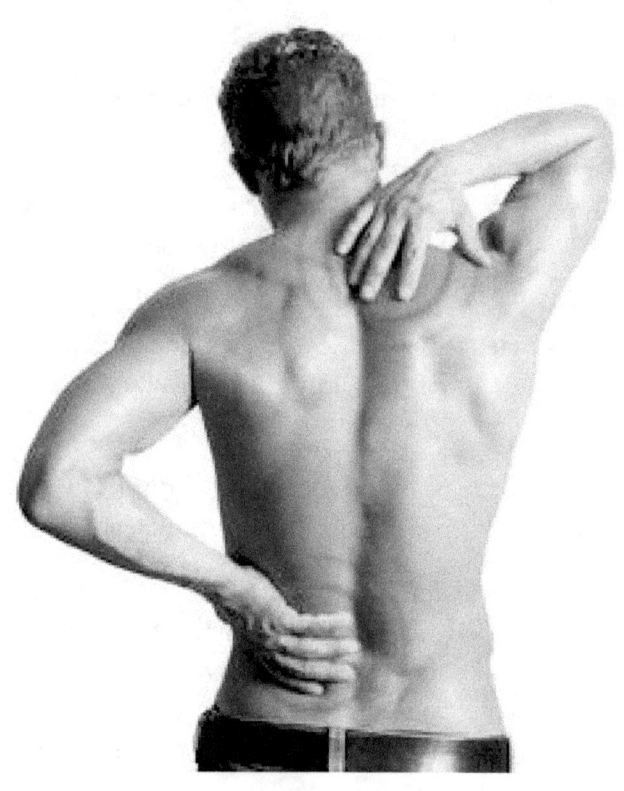

There are plenty of traditional remedies available for you out there, especially over the counter remedies. However, if the plan is really severe, you may want to consult the doctor right now so that he can give you painkillers. Remember a precise and early diagnosis of arthritis can prevent any irreversible damage.

Massage is a good way in which the joints can be kept supple and active. However, only your doctor can tell you if you have arthritis, or any related condition and what you need to do about it. Do not keep waiting for the pain to go away because it can get aggravated.

Risk Factors for Arthritis

The common risk factors for arthritis, especially some of which can be controlled, and some which are unmodifiable are given below.

Risk factors – Non– modifiable

These risk factors are going to consist of age, gender and genetic tendency towards arthritis. The risk of developing any type of arthritis increases as you grow older.

There are specific genes, which are associated with a higher risk of certain types of arthritis. These genes can cause rheumatoid arthritis, ankylosing spondylitis, and systemic lupus erythematosus. So if you are genetically prone to these arthritis types, there is a chance that you are going to suffer from that as you grow older.

Most types of arthritis are more common in women. On the other hand, men are more prone to gout. This takes the form of inflammation of the foot, especially the toes. This is called gout.

Gout was once considered to be the scourge of the aristocracy, especially in the 18th and 19th century, because that was the time when they definitely were not moderate in their diet.

They drank and ate in copious quantities, especially plenty of red meat and drinking wine, Stout, and other alcoholic beverages, which aggravated the gouty condition.

Thus diet is one risk factor, which can be modified. Elevated uric acid levels in your body are going to lead to gout. These high uric acid levels are caused due to eating food items like red meat and less of vegetables and fruit.

Excess weight can also contribute to the progression and onset of osteoarthritis of the knee. That is because the legs have to carry the weight of the upper body.

Infections are also a modifiable risk factor, which can potentially lead to arthritis. If your joints have been infected by bacteria and viruses, especially because of low immunity, this is going to cause the development of different forms of arthritis.

Injuries to your joints, especially the knee and the hips can also lead to potential arthritis.

Preventive measures for arthritis

Did you know that bending regularly can also contribute to osteoarthritis of the knee? And here you were thinking, that this was the best way in which you could keep your muscles and joints limber. You need to find the right balance between rest and activity.

Exercising too much may stress sensitive joints. On the same principle a too sedentary lifestyle can cause more immobility and stiffness. In fact, people like I and you, who spend a lot of time sitting right in front of the computer are going to prevent osteoarthritis from striking, by getting up occasionally and taking small and frequent walks.

You may try a gentle movements and stretching exercises such as those done by yoga, which are easy to the joints. They are going to keep them supple and fluid.

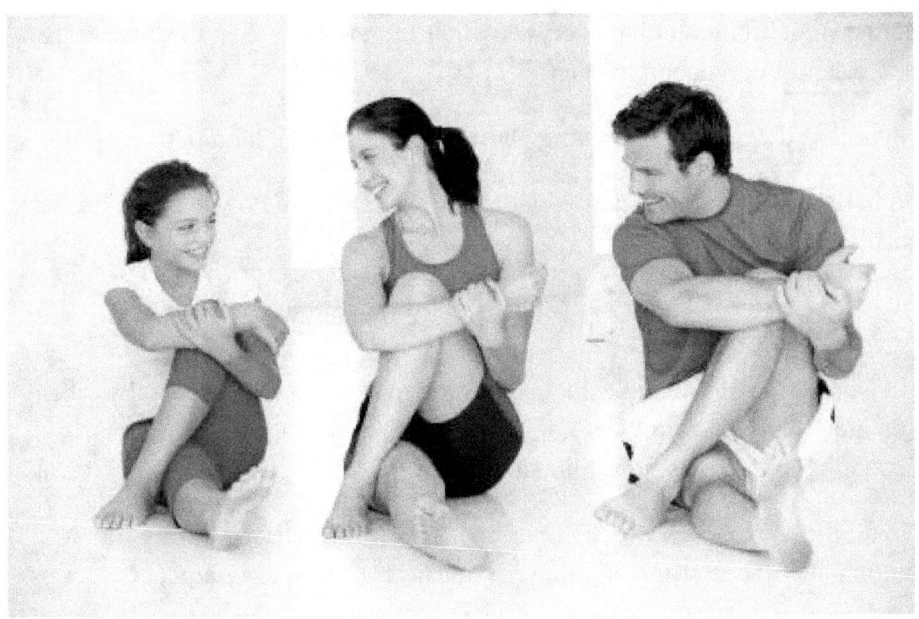

Yoga, started young can keep you healthy and fit throughout your life. Make sure your body does not suffer from any sort of stress and strain, when you are doing any sort of exercise routine, including yoga.

Some well-known exercises, aerobics, especially those done in water and riding a bike can keep the muscles of your body strong, and your heart healthy. But they put too much pressure on the joints so I would suggest not doing these joints stressing exercises, if you suffer from severe joint pain.

I remember one of the doctors I knew telling a patient who was suffering from arthritis in many to do a little bit of jogging and running. I happen to be there, and I said that this should be avoided, because that would put pressure on his knee. I still remember that nasty glare given to me by the doctor, because of course he knew best.

Three months later, that poor man's arthritis condition had worsened so much that he did not know what to do. The running had aggravated the joint inflammation. Of course I did not tell him I told you so, because he would have taken the nearest chair and placed a juicy one upon my head, if I did, but he went around telling everybody that I knew more than the doctor. But this was just plain common sense.

Naturally, the doctor has put me on his blacklist as blabbermouth enemies!

So here are the do's and don'ts which you are going to do when you are suffering from arthritis.

Do's

Here are some of the do's which are going to come useful, especially when you are looking for ways and means in which to manage arthritis from becoming a severe and disabling ailment.

Do all those exercises which are going to allow muscles to work without putting any undue stress on joints. You can call them low-impact exercises.

Stretching, especially that stretching done, the moment you wake up is going to improve muscle tone. It is also going to help make your joints more supple.

You need to warm up the joints and muscles before you do any sort of stretching exercises. That can be done by doing stationary or non-stationary cycling movements.

Low-impact aerobic exercises along with swimming and walking are good ways to keep your joints and muscles healthy.

Maintain your healthy body weight to reduce stress on these joints, especially those joints which are going to bear all the weight like your hips and your needs.

When you have experienced any sort of joint injury, you need to protect it and allow it to heal properly. Protecting your injured joint now is going to lower the chances of developing arthritis later.

Make sure that that particular joint is not injured again. For example, if you have previously sprained an ankle due to a twisted heel, start wearing flat shoes and throw your heeled shoes away. Use some common sense.

If you are prone to knee injuries, remember that going in for any sort of high-impact physical exercise like football, soccer, volleyball or basketball is not a good idea. Not only are you exposing your body to potential injury, but there is also a chance that you are going to wrench your knee again.

Many a brilliant sporting career has been nipped in the bud, because one ignored an injury to a potentially weak joint. And that led to that particular area being a trouble spot for the rest of the sport man's life.

If you have a particular joint, which is giving you trouble, due to its having being injured, you need to make sure that you do not do any sort of task, which is going to place any sort of strain on that particular region. This is going to prevent you from suffering needless pain, and is also going to help that area heal in its own natural way.

Remember to stop exercising, if you experience any sort of sharp pain. Do not act like a martyr and keep punishing your body in a grueling exercise session just to prove something to yourself or to your trainer, even though your joint is giving you some discomfort. That is only harming your joint even more. Again, use common sense.

You may want to look at activities that are gentle on your body and you need to do them at a very comfortable place, possibly in slow motion.

Make sure that your liquid intake is enough to keep your cartilage in the joints well dehydrated and lubricated. This is going to prevent your bones from rubbing against each other.

If your job requires you to keep standing for a long while, remember to take some time off after every half an hour, and set your muscles moving. A person with joints problem can never be a guard standing outside Buckingham Palace!

Don'ts

These are the don'ts which you need to follow.

Long walking, running and jogging is strictly forbidden, especially as these activities can only be done by people who have healthy joint muscles.

Weightlifting, especially when you have aching joints is not advisable. Also, do not sit cross legged, because that is going to put stress on your hipbones, and on your knees.

Also, climbing stairs, especially when you are suffering from joint problems should be avoided. That is because we have the bad habit of putting all our weight on our feet, when we go up or go downstairs. Every single step is going to have an impact, felt through the soles of our feet right onto that affected joint, especially if it is in the knee.

Diet

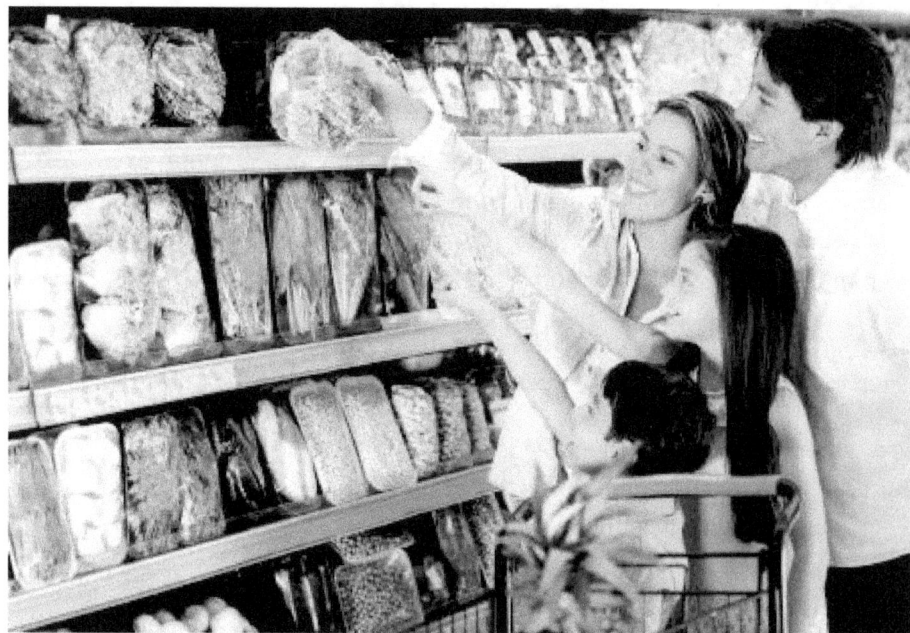

Is there any particular diet, which is going to help prevent and cure arthritis? Well, common sense says that any food which is going to cause an inflammation to flare up needs to be avoided. This includes red meat and alcohol. Instead, you may want to add more fruits and vegetables to your diet.

Start eating fish, especially omega 3 rich fish like salmon, mackerel, trout, tuna and sardines. If you do not want to eat fish, you can eat soybeans and walnuts.

Olive oil and whole grains are also excellent to keep your system healthy.

Natural Cures for Arthritis

Tomatoes

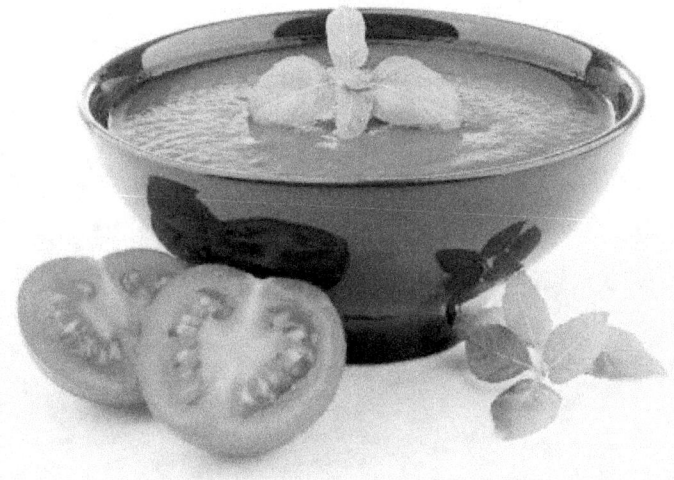

Tomatoes are considered to be good for the heart, because they contain nicotinic acid. They are believed to reduce cholesterol and vitamin K content in the tomatoes is an anti-hemorrhagic.

Tomatoes have long been used as an antiseptic, as well as a preventative food against infections for millenniums.

Lots of tomato juice drunk regularly means that you are going to have a natural blood purifier, getting into your system. Tomato juice is also well known to be an excellent healer for natural therapeutic treatment of arthritis.

Thyme Tea

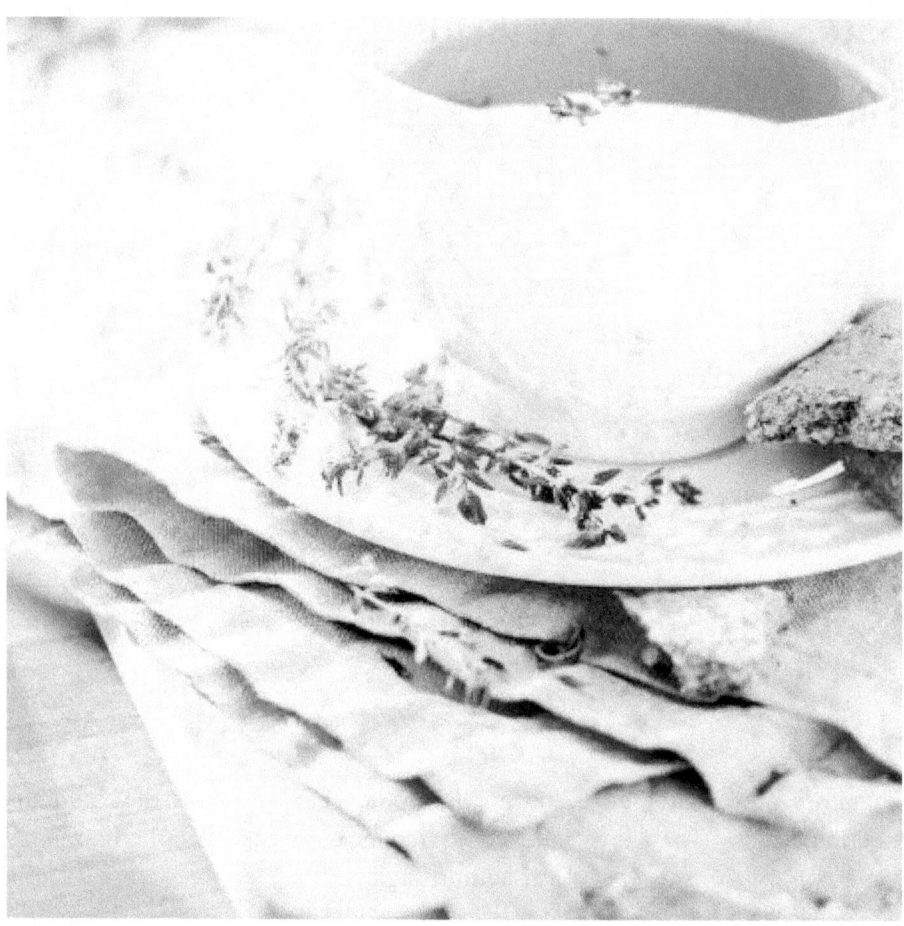

This tea is an herbal remedy, given to people suffering from insomnia. A herbal tea infusion is going to be made up of one teaspoonful of dried herb, in a glass of boiling hot water. Allow it to infuse for 15 minutes and then drink. No nightmares when you sleep tonight.

This tea is excellent for arthritis too.

This tea should not be given to ladies who are expecting. In fact, if they stop eating thyme, especially its seeds all through their pregnancy, it is going to be healthier for the baby.

This is also excellent for a person suffering from colic and flatulence.

Massage Treatment for Arthritis

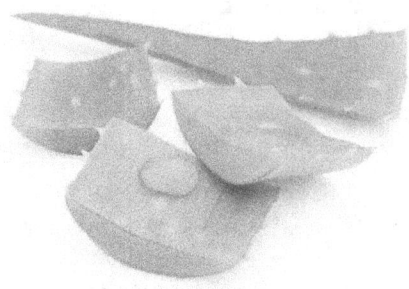

You use Aloe Vera here. Treat arthritis by massaging a mixture of Aloe Vera pulp in warm mustard oil, all over the affected area. You can also extract the pulp, heat it with any oil – coconut oil, wheat germ oil and olive oil – place it on a piece of cotton and allow it to "foment" the painful area. This is going to alleviate the pain.

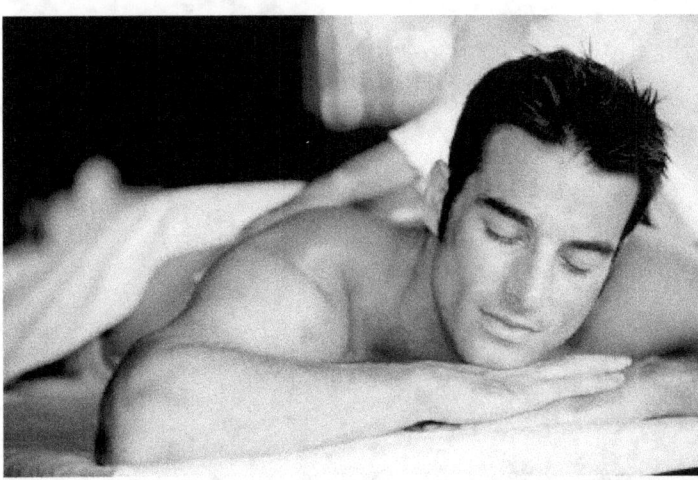

It is not necessary for you to suffer from any sort of joint pain in order to enjoy a massage. Since ancient times, massaging with aromatic and healing oils has been a good way to keep the system moving well, the skin looking healthy and youthful and the muscles growing in good condition.

Thyme oil – Arthritis Remedy

Use original thyme oil for massaging all the affected parts, while you are drinking thyme tea, made by steeping half a teaspoonful of dried thyme, in a glass of water, water, and allowing to infuse for 20 minutes.

In the East, this oil was used on summer afternoons, for massaging the affected areas, especially for old people to make the muscles more supple, and to prevent the joints from stiffening up during arthritis.

Thyme oil needs to be bought in its natural form. *Do not buy thymol*, which is the chemical equivalent and definitely does not have the hundred percent natural qualities.

It may come a bit expensive, but if you know a place where you can get this oil, especially in organic and aromatherapy stores, you do not have to worry about arthritis anymore.

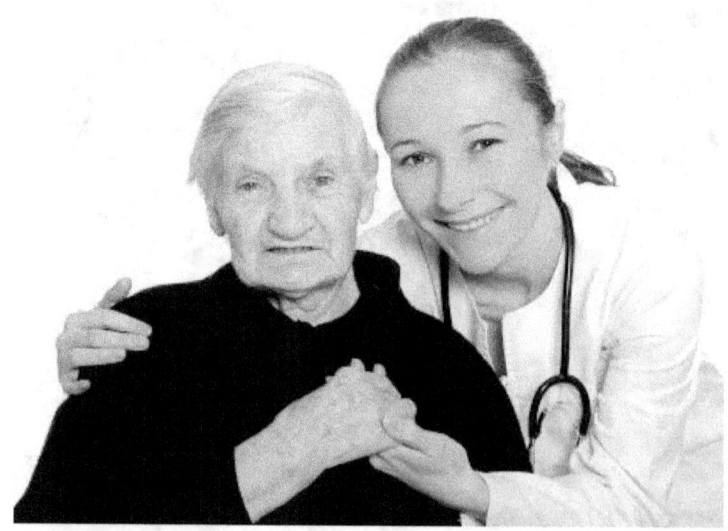

Regular massaging with thyme oil means she does not have to worry about arthritis pain or even joint pains.

You can either use it in small quantities, either on its own, or you can mix it up with another good massaging oil like coconut, mustard or olive oil a little warmed up so that it can get better absorbed in the muscular tissue.

In ancient times, this massage was done every day, to anybody who could be caught, be they man, woman or child. That is because this loosened the muscles, and in the case of children, this encouraged muscular growth. It also kept the skin glowing and healthy.

Treating Gout

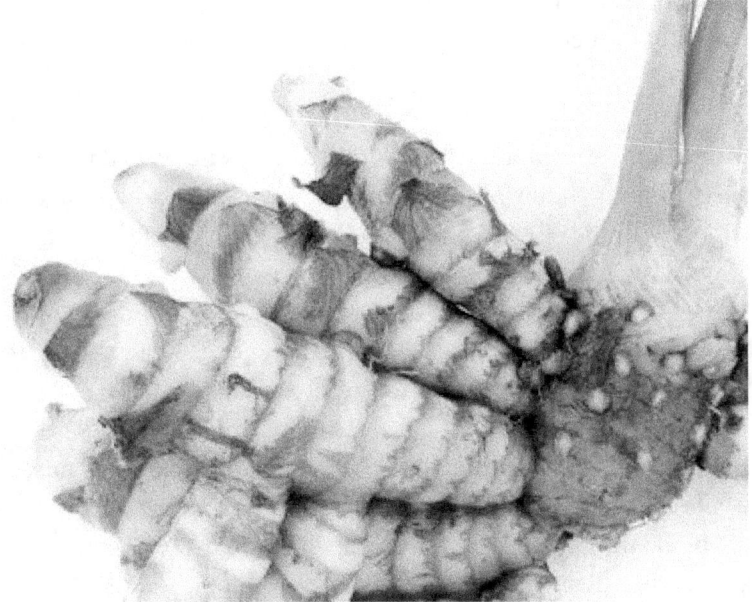

Arthritis is basically an autoimmune disorder which affects your joints. Gout is the building up of uric acid crystals in a particular area, which makes that area swollen, along with purple, hot and swollen joints.

You need 25 g of dried ginger for making this gout remedy. Fry it in sesame oil until the ginger turns brown. I am suggesting sesame oil, because it does not sting – and stink – too much. The original traditional gout remedy was made in clarified butter, which is prohibitively expensive now, but at that time was plentiful in the East. Those who did not have clarified butter around used mustard oil. And mustard oil is another stinker, literally.

Now sieve the ginger oil and bottle it in a glass bottle. Massage the affected areas with this oil, especially on the joints. This is supposed to make the joints supple.
Also, the herbalist who told me this remedy told me that one needed to fry 10 g of ginger in Clarified Butter made from cow's milk. That made the system healthy and alleviated the pain due to gout.

This worked wonders for arthritis and painful joints, because gout is normally limited to a painful toe and painful joints.

My father who is in his 80s, told me that this ginger oil remedy was used for massaging the limbs of the old people in his ancestral village and anyone who died at the age of 95 was said to have died young! Many of them crossed the hundred years mark.

So I think that there is something in good genes , a healthy diet and living in healthy natural surroundings to promote longevity.

He also said that after they had got a massage done with mustard oil, they went out in groups to have a vigorous bout of wrestling. The idea was to get the blood moving, before they jumped in the nearest water source to rub off all that dirt, dust, grime and oil.

This helped keep the bones healthy and the joints supple. It also gave the youngsters sleek, well moisturized and good-looking skins! And this suppleness in the bones and in the joints as well as the good looks of the skins persisted until they grew old, with absolutely no worry about joint problems, gout or arthritis.

The longevity and the supple joints of these very active old people can also be due to three reasons – they never sat down and brooded, they just worked and moved around all day long. Like he does from five in the morning to nine thirty at night,- with half an hour's siesta in the afternoons- when he decides that it is time to rest after a day's good physical activities, just pottering around the place!

Also, their diet included proteins, homemade butter and clarified butter. The third thing was if they did not have sesame oil, – especially for joint pains – they used mustard oil, which everybody in the Northern area of the Indian sub-continent considers to be one of the most powerful of massaging oils.

Like I said before it stings and stinks, but unrefined mustard oil is considered to be second to none for keeping your muscles supple, healthy and well-toned.

Also, here comes another secret. My grandmother said that her grandmother, and those who went before her, used to add one red-hot chili pepper to the dried ginger before she "burnt" it. This would make anyone yelp because both of them sting like Billy- O., so you need to use in moderation but the long-term effects to cure joint pain were miraculous.

When we were kids, we were caught by any Elder, who found us floating around and subjected to thorough mustard oil massages, before we were allowed to bake in the sun for half an hour and then scrubbed in a cold bath until we glowed.

This ancient practice is still being followed in many parts of the world, where children are massaged every day so that their limbs grow up to be healthy, strong and straight.

Well, as far I know, this worked for us, because we never suffered from any weak limbs and bones, and got used to using our legs extensively to get our joints working properly, as children and as adults.

QED. Unfortunately, this tradition is going out of practice, because a majority of the mothers of today consider this oiling and massaging a child's limbs to be a thoroughly uncivilized, savage, and barbaric practice. They would not want to indulge in the usage of any sort of oil, which brings out the neighborhood, protesting against the strong aroma.

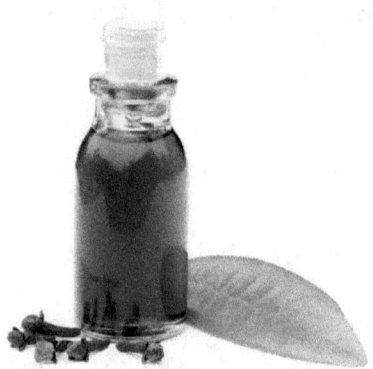

Essential oils have been in use for centuries to help cure ailments, through massage.

Nevertheless, if you want to know all about traditional oil, which was used in the massaging of the limbs of old people, suffering from joint pain, arthritis and other muscle and joint related problems, here it is, given below. You are not going to use it on children. Children should be massaged with warm olive oil or sesame oil or mustard oil, without any herbs and spices added to it.

Traditional Cayenne Hot Oil

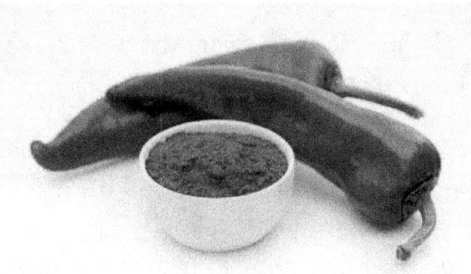

Herbalists know all about the heating and the cooling power of different herbs and spices. So when do you use heating oils? If you are feeling too cold, stiff, chilled, and also, if some portions of your body are cold and stiff, especially in cases like arthritis, then you use a hot oil made up of cayenne. It is going to bring warmth to your body.

This is the special chilli hot oil, which is used traditionally in the East to heal patients in the winter by massaging the affected areas with a little bit of this oil once or twice a day, depending on the severity of the case. You can use them for spasms, cold areas, improving circulation, cramps, muscular aches and chilblains. Also, if you are chilled to the bone, this chilli oil is best for you, no pun intended.

Take these ingredients –

25 g cayenne pepper
2 inches ginger root
2 tablespoons mustard powder.
1/1 x 4 cups vegetable oil- I am using coconut oil here.
2 teaspoons ground black pepper
This is originally made in mustard oil, but because mustard oil has a very strong aroma, I am substituting coconut oil. Coconut oil is equally powerful and equally aromatic, but somehow it is more popular with people in the West.

You can prepare this oil in two ways. One is in the summer, when you can put all the ingredients in a bottle filled with oil. Place the bottle in the sun and allow to infuse in the summer heat for about two months. Shake this glass bottle regularly.

But if winter is already here, and you were too busy to make this infusion in the summer, do this the other way.

Put the dried ginger, and the chilli in half of the oil in a container with a tight lid. Put this container in a pan with lid. Fill the pan with water up to 2 inches from the top. Allow it to simmer slowly for about two hours. Do not heat the oil directly because it is going to be burnt. That is why it has to be done through boiling in water.

Allow this mixture to cool. Now add the rest of the spices to the oil, and stir vigorously. Add the rest of the oil and return to the boiling water pan. Add more water to make sure that there is no dearth of it. Two more hours of slow boiling is going to give you a red colored very powerful infused oil. I would suggest you filter it, because any sort of sediment at the bottom of the oil is going to spoil it.

Collect those spices. You may use them in cooking or if you want or you may add some more spices to them, and some more oil, and put them outside in the sun for more infused oil by next summer!

You may find some sediment settling down at the bottom of the pan, after about three months. Remove that sediment or watery liquid which may just be parts of herbs which were not filtered, initially, appearing to settle down at the bottom of the bottle. This is going to spoil the oily if it is not removed.

Remember that the cold months of winter does not mean that you need to suffer. Use a little bit of this oil to massage those aching joints and pains.

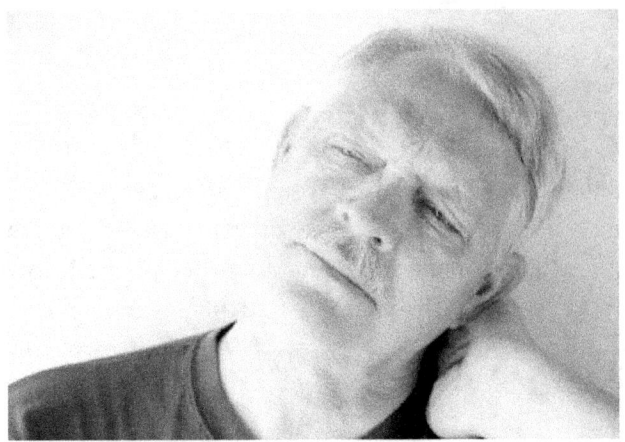

No joint pain ever again with a hot oil rub.

Fennel Seeds for Arthritis

Fennel is excellent as a diuretic. It prevents water retention. So just drink it as a tea, or just eat the seeds as often as you can. Also, if you are suffering from arthritis, just try adding a little quantity of fennel seeds to your daily diet. You are soon going to see an improvement.

Olive Oil Cure

Warm some olive oil. Add the juice of a lemon in this warm oil, and gently massage the affected part with this oil for half an hour. Now bandage that massaged area and leave overnight. The next morning, drink 1 tablespoon full of cider vinegar and 1 tablespoon full of honey in a glass of lukewarm water. This is going to do wonders for your arthritis

Is Surgery Advisable?

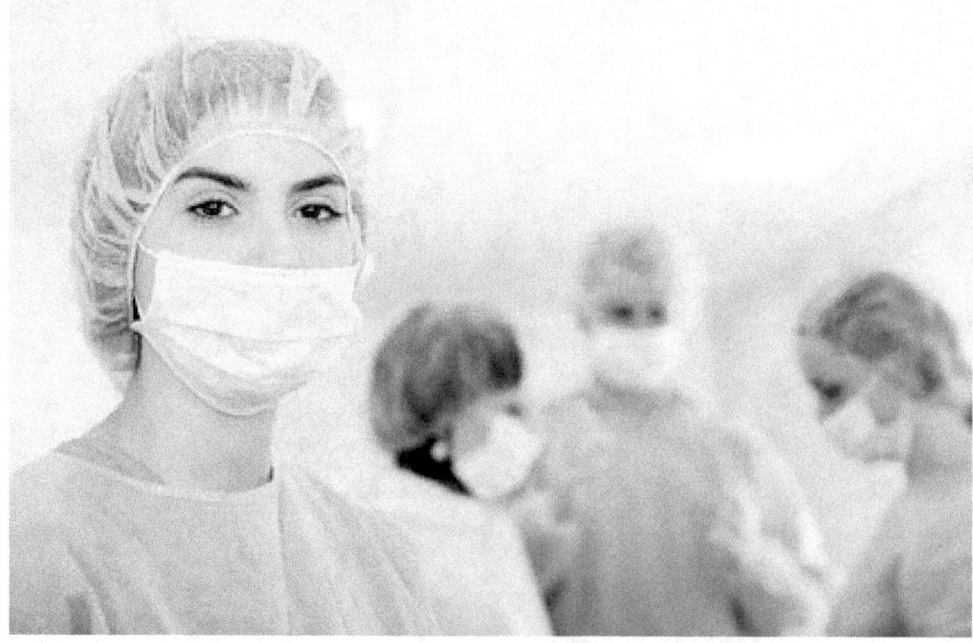

Did you know that many doctors are prescribing immediate surgery for advanced stages of arthritis? Today, every patient wants an accurate and less invasive surgery method so that he can return back to his normal lifestyle easily and quickly.

Many of the surgical processes advised today include joint replacement. But how necessary is it? That depends on the severity of your condition.

State-of-the-art surgical processes allow minimally invasive surgeries with the least amount of pain, blood loss, and gaining of flexibility, almost like a natural knee, especially in matters of knee surgery.

Do I recommend surgical procedures? Well, it depends on you whether you can afford it, and the doctor recommends it for you.

According to one of the surgeons who was discussing the concept of knee replacement surgery with me, he said that state-of-the-art knee replacement which lasts more than 30 years is a concept beyond an implant.

It was a complex combination of high quality bio – materials, alignment, accuracy gender specific design, technology and sizing. This would give a biological need a replacement with high bending and longevity of more than 30 years.

99% accurate results have been obtained in many large hospitals, especially those hospitals which help a patient suffering from knee joint problems lead a much more active life.

Many of these patients find it difficult in doing such a day to day activities like walking on uneven surfaces, climbing upstairs, rising from a low seat, kneeling, and even bending down.

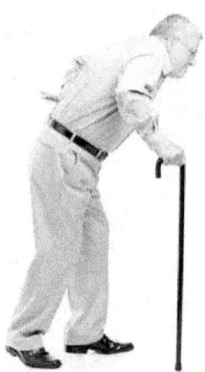

CAS – Computer Assisted Knee Surgery

Computer assisted surgery can allow a surgeon to align the patient's bones and the joint implants with an astonishing degree of accuracy, which is normally not possible with the naked eye.

The key benefits of such a surgery means that this minimally invasive process is going to offer the potential for faster recovery, lesser damage to the bone and tissue, and lesser pain.

The natural restoration of your anatomy when compared to a conventional total knee replacement is thus going to be done with this surgical process.

Pinless Computer Navigation

Pinless computer navigation, is far less invasive when compared with CAS. No incision is going to be made in the thigh bone or in the shinbone.

This means that the risk of infection is drastically reduced. That means your new knee is going to last for a longer period of time.

There are plenty of specialized hospitals all over the world, giving you the best solutions for healing through expensive surgical processes. If your doctor recommends this process for you, and you can afford it, you may want to look at this option, especially if you are suffering from a very severe case of knee joint inflammation.

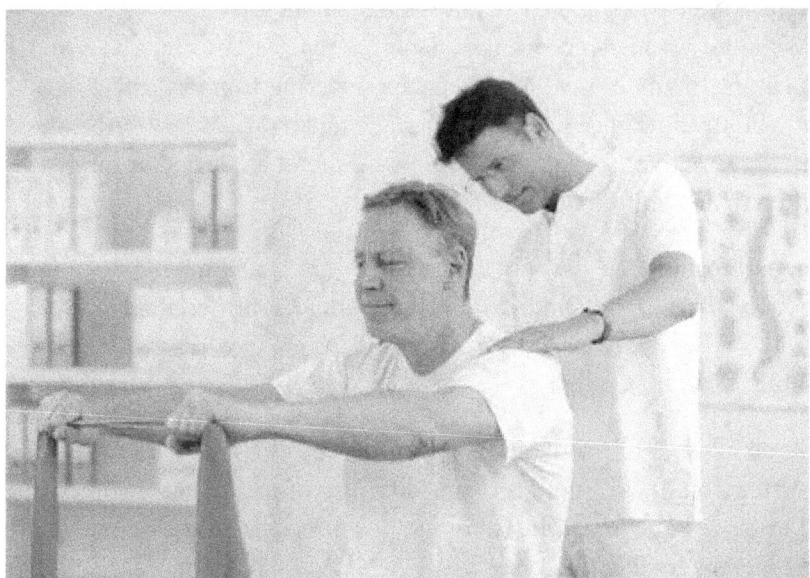

Conclusion

This book has given you some basic knowledge about arthritis, its symptoms, and how you can prevent it. Doctors say that it cannot be cured. Frankly speaking, many of my acquaintances suffering from arthritis are managing to control it rather well with massage and a proper diet. Also they remember to stay active, though they make sure that that particular joint is not submitted to any sort of stress or tension.

Arthritis in any form is one particular ailment, which many people do not know as begun to claim the number one slot among health problems in many parts of the world, overtaking serious conditions like heart ailments, cancer, diabetes and hypertension.

In fact, a large number of people in the age group of 40 – 45 years have begun to suffer from these joint problems, because of negligence or accidental trauma to the joints, inflammation of infected muscles, tissue and bones and other such allied factors.

So if you are suffering from any sort of joint problem, which causes you pain, and stiffness, it could either be arthritis, or it could be another associated or unrelated potentially serious and chronic problem.

Do not neglect it. Get your doctor to do a proper checkup and then give you the best advice so that this ailment can be managed before it causes any sort of irreversible damage and disability to your body.

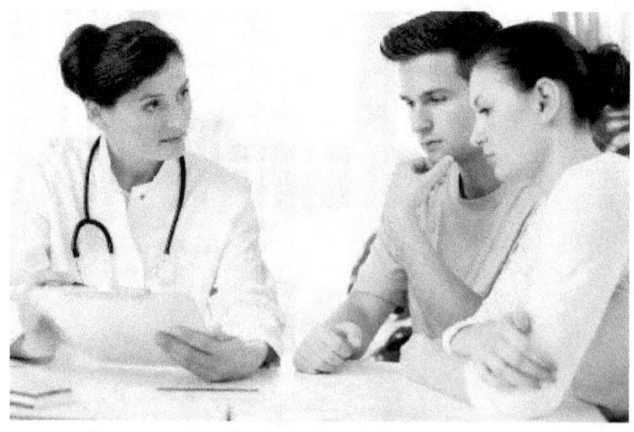

Proper medical advice taken at the right time can prevent you from suffering from future ailments, including arthritis.

Live Long and Prosper!

Author Bio

Dueep Jyot Singh is a Management and IT Professional who managed to gather Postgraduate qualifications in Management and English and Degrees in Science, French and Education while pursuing different enjoyable career options like being an hospital administrator, IT,SEO and HRD Database Manager/ trainer, movie , radio and TV scriptwriter, theatre artiste and public speaker, lecturer in French, Marketing and Advertising, ex-Editor of Hearts On Fire (now known as Solstice) Books Missouri USA, advice columnist and cartoonist, publisher and Aviation School trainer, ex-moderator on Medico.in, banker, student councilor ,travelogue writer … among other things!

One fine morning, she decided that she had enough of killing herself by Degrees and went back to her first love -- writing. It's more enjoyable! She already has 48 published academic and 14 fiction- in- different- genre books under her belt.

When she is not designing websites or making Graphic design illustrations for clients , she is browsing through old bookshops hunting for treasures, of which she has an enviable collection – including R.L. Stevenson, O.Henry, Dornford Yates, Maurice Walsh, De Maupassant, Victor Hugo, Sapper, C.N. Williamson, "Bartimeus" and the crown of her collection- Dickens "The Old Curiosity Shop," and so on… Just call her "Renaissance Woman") - collecting herbal remedies, acting like Universal Helping Hand/Agony Aunt, or escaping to her dear mountains for a bit of exploring, collecting herbs and plants and trekking.

Check out some of the other JD-Biz Publishing books

Gardening Series on Amazon

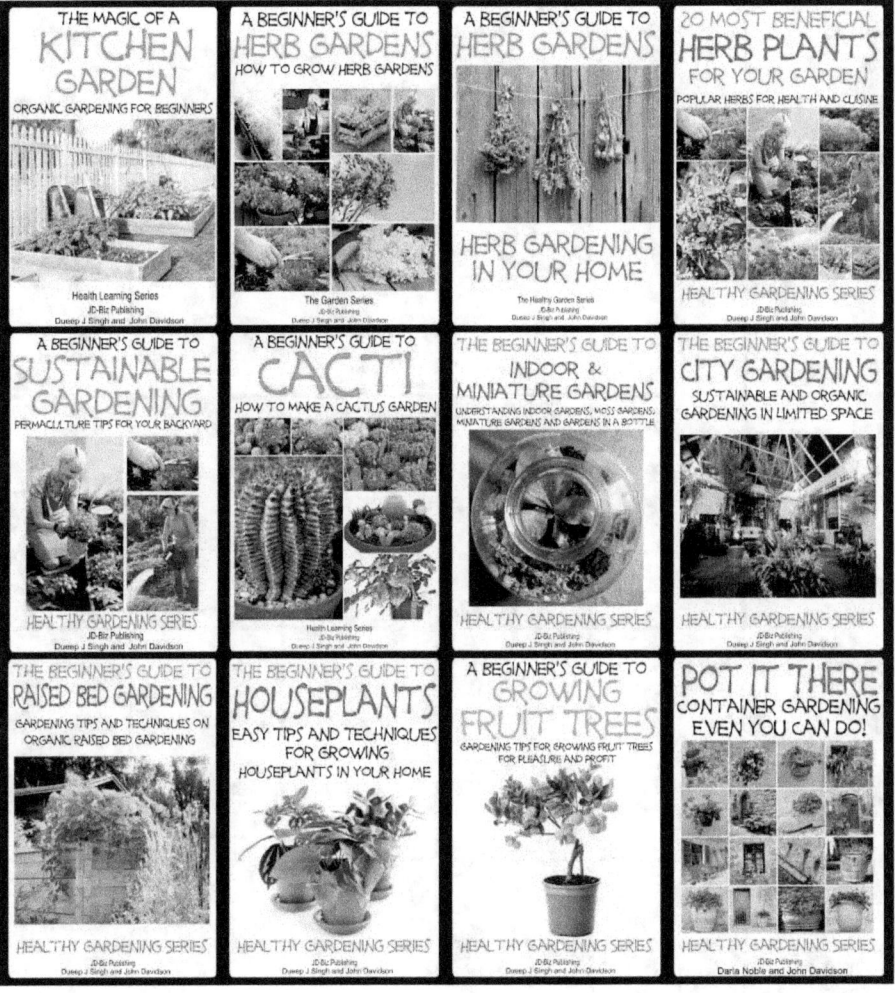

THE MAGIC OF GOOSEBERRIES FOR HEALTH AND BEAUTY — Natural Remedy Series

THE MAGIC OF YOGURT FOR COOKING AND BEAUTY — Natural Remedy Series

THE MAGIC OF LEMONS USING LEMONS FOR HEALTH AND BEAUTY — Natural Remedy Series

THE MAGIC OF CHILLIES FOR COOKING AND HEALING — Natural Remedy Series

THE MAGIC OF ONIONS ONIONS IN CUISINE TO CURE AND TO HEAL — Natural Remedy Series

THE MAGIC OF RADISHES TO CURE AND TO HEAL — Natural Remedy Series

THE MAGIC OF CARROTS TO CURE AND TO HEAL — Natural Remedy Series

THE HEALTH BENEFITS OF OREGANO FOR COOKING AND HEALTH — Natural Remedy Series

The Magic Of MARIGOLDS Marigolds for Health And Beauty — Natural Remedy Series

THE HEALTH BENEFITS OF CINNAMON — Natural Remedy Series

THE MAGIC OF COCONUTS FOR COOKING & HEALTH — Health Learning Series

THE MAGIC OF CLOVES FOR HEALING AND COOKING — Health Learning Series

THE MAGIC OF ASAFETIDA FOR COOKING AND HEALING — Health Learning Series

THE MAGIC OF NEEM MARGOSA TO HEAL — Natural Remedy Series

THE MAGIC OF SALT TO HEAL AND FOR BEAUTY — Natural Remedy Series

THE MAGIC OF POMEGRANATES FOR HEALTH AND BEAUTY — Natural Remedy Series

THE MAGIC OF DRY FRUIT AND SPICES REMEDIES AND RECIPES — Natural Remedy Series

THE HEALTH BENEFITS OF TURMERIC CURCUMIN FOR COOKING AND HEALTH — Natural Remedy Series

THE MAGIC OF ALOE VERA — Natural Remedy Series

THE MAGIC OF VEGETABLES ANCIENT HEALING REMEDIES AND TIPS — Natural Remedy Series

THE HEALTH BENEFITS OF ROSEMARY FOR COOKING AND HEALTH — Natural Remedy Series

THE MAGIC OF PEPPER & PEPPERCORNS FOR COOKING & HEALING — Natural Remedy Series

THE MAGIC OF MILK, BUTTER AND CHEESE FOR COOKING & HEALING — Natural Remedy Series

THE MAGIC OF CARDAMOMS FOR COOKING AND HEALTH — Health Learning Series

THE HEALTH BENEFITS OF BLACK CUMIN FOR COOKING AND HEALTH — Natural Remedy Series

THE MAGIC OF BASIL-TULSI TO HEAL NATURALLY — Health Learning Series

THE MAGIC OF SPICES FOR HEALTH AND CUISINE — Natural Remedy Series

THE MAGIC OF ROSES FOR COOKING AND BEAUTY — Natural Remedy Series

The Miraculous Healing Powers of GINGER — Natural Remedy Series — BEST

The Miracle of HONEY — Natural Remedy Series — BEST

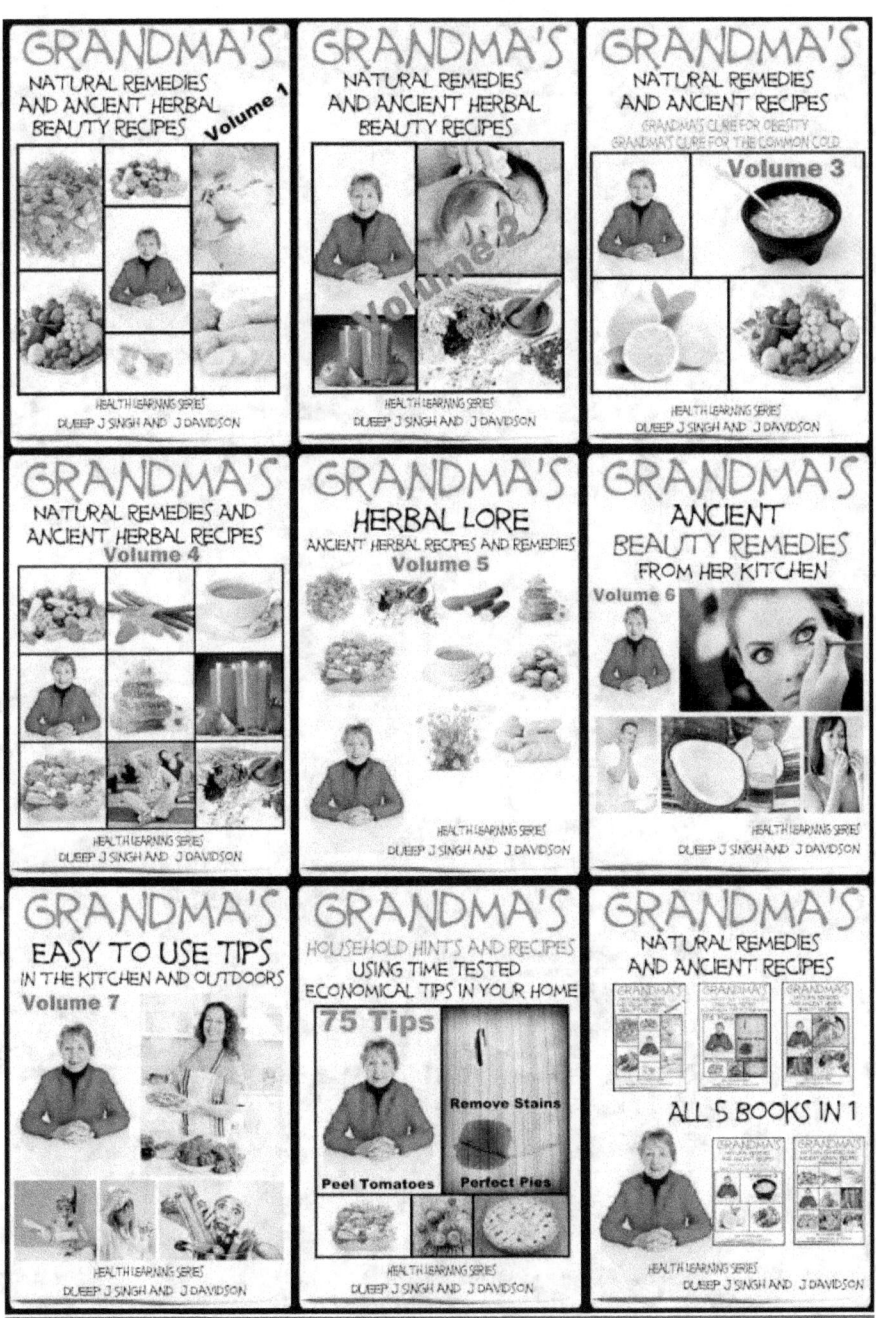

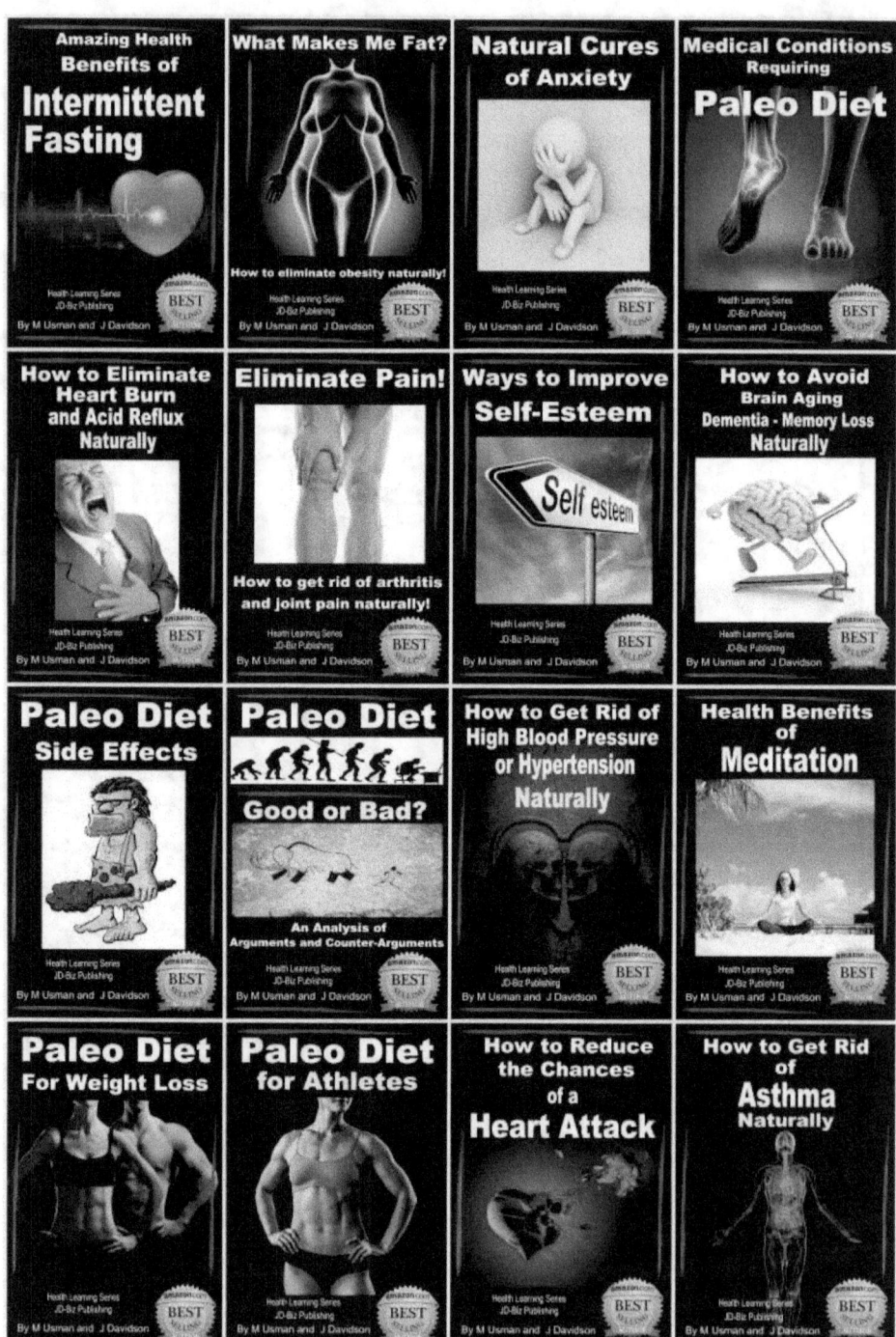

Amazing Animal Book Series

Learn To Draw Series

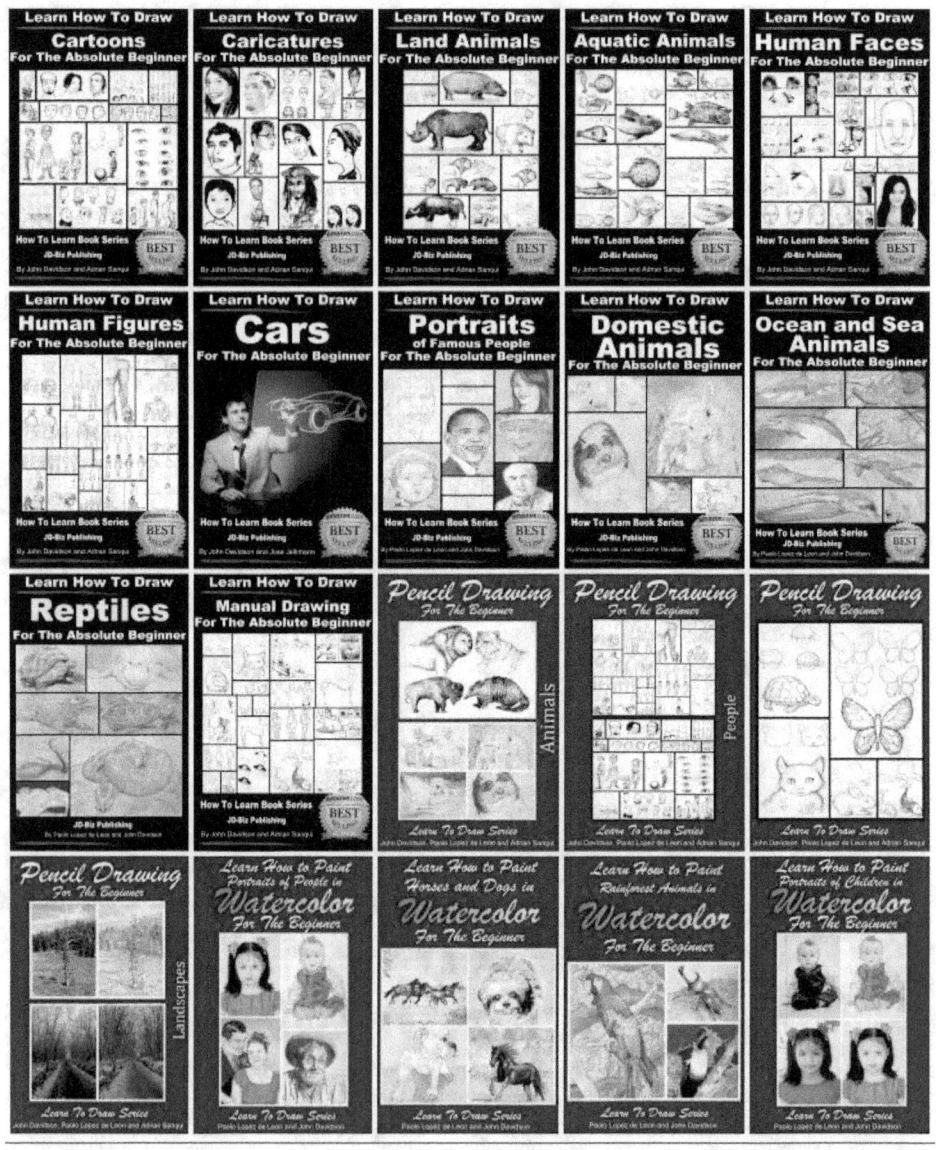

How to Build and Plan Books

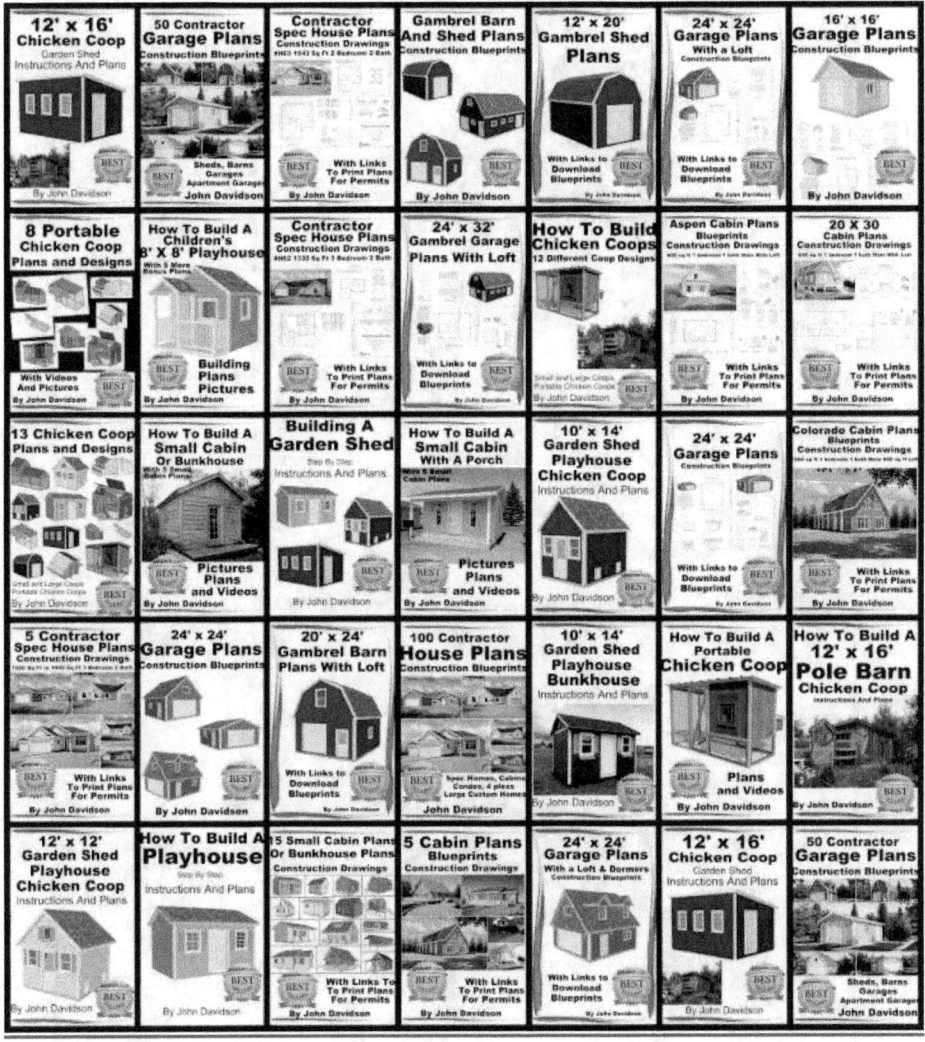

Entrepreneur Book Series

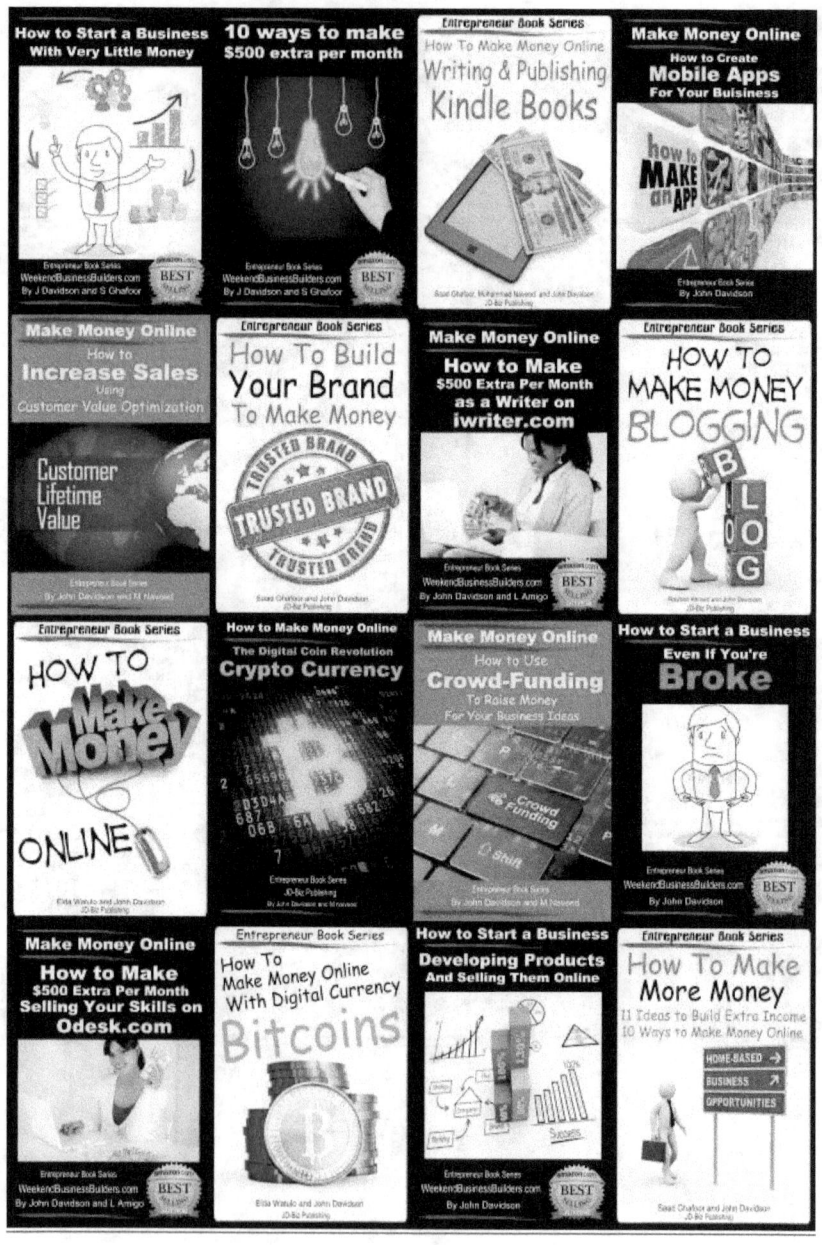

Our books are available at

1. Amazon.com

2. Barnes and Noble

3. Itunes

4. Kobo

5. Smashwords

6. Google Play Books

This book is published by

JD-BIZ
PUBLISHING

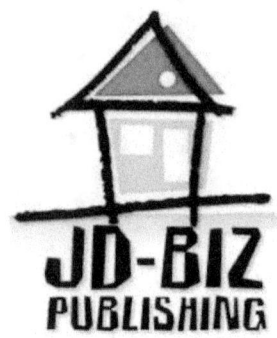

JD-Biz Corp

P O Box 374

Mendon, Utah 84325

http://www.jd-biz.com/

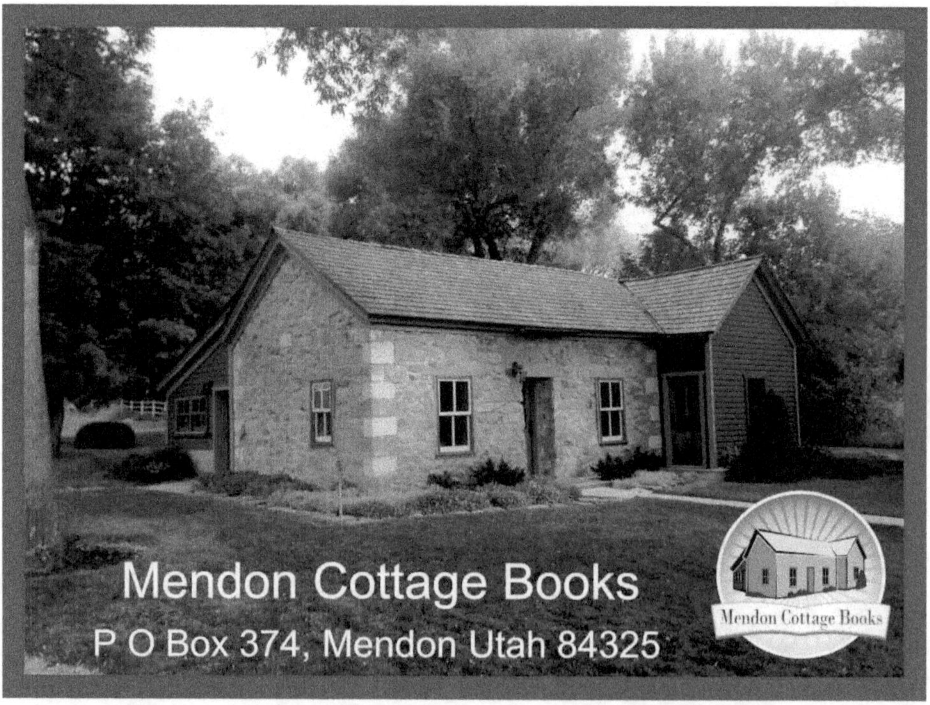

Mendon Cottage Books
P O Box 374, Mendon Utah 84325
Mendon Cottage Books

www.ingramcontent.com/pod-product-compliance
Lightning Source LLC
Chambersburg PA
CBHW061928280526
45787CB00004B/1526